Plant-Based Soups, Salads & More

An Innovative Cookbook for Perfect Meals

Lily Mullen

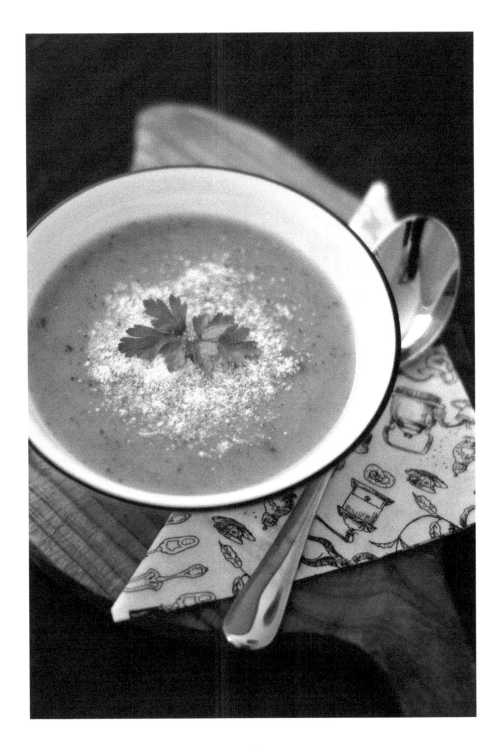

TABLE OF CONTENTS

Introduction

A plant-based eating routine backing and upgrades the entirety of this. For what reason should most of what we eat originate from the beginning?

Eating more plants is the first nourishing convention known to man to counteract and even turn around the ceaseless diseases that assault our general public.

Plants and vegetables are brimming with large scale and micronutrients that give our bodies all that we require for a sound and productive life. By eating, at any rate, two suppers stuffed with veggies consistently, and nibbling on foods grown from the ground in the middle of, the nature of your wellbeing and at last your life will improve.

The most widely recognized wellbeing worries that individuals have can be reduced by this one straightforward advance.

Things like weight, inadequate rest, awful skin, quickened maturing, irritation, physical torment, and absence of vitality would all be able to be decidedly influenced by expanding the admission of plants and characteristic nourishments.

If you're reading this book, then you're probably on a journey to get healthy because you know good health and nutrition go hand in hand.

Maybe you're looking at the plant-based diet as a solution to those love handles.

Whatever the case may be, the standard American diet millions of people eat daily is not the best way to fuel your body.

If you ask me, any other diet will already be a significant improvement. Since what you eat fuels your body, you can imagine that eating junk will make you feel just that—like junk.

I've followed the standard American diet for several years: my plate was loaded with high-fat and carbohydrate-rich foods. I know this doesn't sound like a horrible way to eat, but keep in mind that most Americans don't focus on eating healthy fats and complex carbs—we live on processed foods.

The consequences of eating foods filled with trans fats, preservatives, and mountains of sugar are fatigue, reduced mental focus, mood swings, and weight gain. To top it off, there's the issue of opening yourself up to certain diseases— some life-threatening—when you neglect paying attention to what you eat .

Zucchini Balsamic Vinegar Burgers

Preparation time: 10 minutes

Cooking time: 50 minutes

Servings 4–6 burgers

Ingredients:

- 1 zucchini, cut in 1/4 inch thick slices
- 2 tablespoons olive oil
- 1 tablespoon balsamic vinegar
- Salt, pepper

Directions:

1. To take the bitterness out of zucchini, there is a simple process.
2. Place the zucchini slices in a colander and sprinkle slices with an ample amount of salt.
3. Leave the zucchini with salt in colander for thirty minutes.
4. Rinse the zucchini and dab them dry with paper towels.

5. Place in mixing bowl, drizzle olive oil over slices and toss until evenly coated.
6. Add one tablespoon of olive oil to frying pan and heat over medium.
7. Cook burgers on each side 4 minutes, until golden in color.
8. Remove from heat and soak in balsamic vinegar, salt and pepper.
9. Serve delicious slices over your favorite choice of bread and toppings.

Tofu Portobello Burgers

Preparation time: 10 minutes

Cooking time: 60 minutes

Servings 4 burgers

Ingredients:

- 4 Portobello mushrooms
- 1 large red onion, sliced
- 1 tablespoon balsamic vinegar
- 2 garlic cloves, minced
- 2 tablespoons olive oil
- 10 oz firm packed tofu
- 1/2 cup red wine
- 1 tablespoon soy sauce
- 1 teaspoon agave syrup
- 1 tablespoon sesame seeds

Directions:

1. In a medium mixing bowl, whisk together the four ingredients below the tofu in the list, include a dash of freshly ground pepper.
2. Slice the tofu and place in mixture for thirty minutes to infuse with flavor.
3. Prepare the portabellas for cooking by slicing and removing stems.
4. Fry the mushrooms over medium heat until cooked through.
5. Remove mushrooms and place tofu in same pan.
6. Cook until browned.
7. Mix together the remaining ingredients.
8. Layer ingredients and marinade over bread and serve.

Chickpeas Burgers

Preparation time: 10 minutes

Cooking time: 40 minutes

Servings 6–8 burgers

Ingredients:

- 3 oz bulgur
- 2 cups water
- 1 1/2 cups canned chickpeas
- 1/2 cup fresh chopped parsley
- 1 tablespoon all purpose flour
- 2 garlic cloves, minced
- 2 tablespoons breadcrumbs
- 1 tablespoon olive oil
- Salt, pepper (to taste)

Directions:

1. Bring 2 cups water to a boil.
2. Add bulgur and cook until water has been absorbed, let cool.

3. Create a paste with the chickpeas by placing in food processor and pulsing.
4. Add the paste and remaining ingredient list to the bulgur and combine.
5. Using wet hands, form the mixture into a burger shape.
6. Add one tablespoon of olive oil to frying pan and heat over medium.
7. Cook burgers on each side approximately 5 minutes, until golden brown.

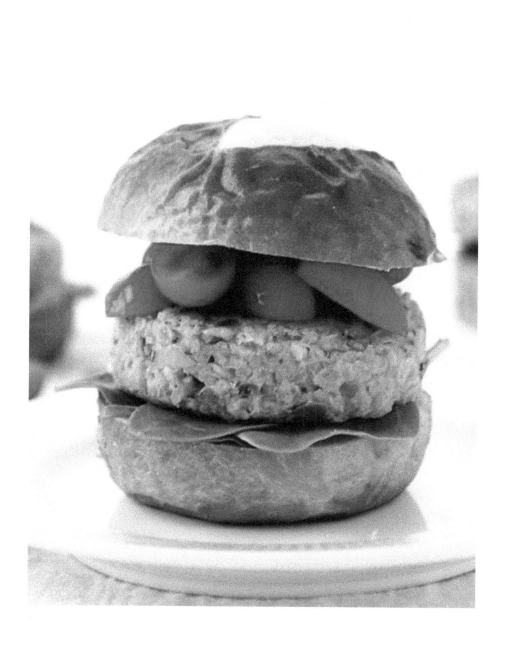

Tomato Eggplant Spinach Salad

Preparation time: 30 minutes

Serves: 4

Ingredients:

- 1 large eggplant, cut into 3/4 inch slices
- 5 oz spinach
- 1 tbsp sun-dried tomatoes, chopped
- 1 tbsp oregano, chopped
- 1 tbsp parsley, chopped
- 1 tbsp fresh mint, chopped
- 1 tbsp shallot, chopped

For dressing:

- 1/4 cup olive oil
- 1/2 lemon juice
- 1/2 tsp smoked paprika
- 1 tsp Dijon mustard
- 1 tsp tahini
- 2 garlic cloves, minced
- Pepper
- Salt

Directions:

1. Place sliced eggplants into the large bowl and sprinkle with salt and set aside for minutes.
2. In a small bowl mix together all dressing ingredients.
3. Set aside.
4. Heat grill to medium-high heat.
5. In a large bowl, add shallot, sun-dried tomatoes, herbs, and spinach.
6. Rinse eggplant slices and pat dry with paper towel.
7. Brush eggplant slices with olive oil and grill on medium high heat for 3-4 minutes on each side.
8. Let cool the grilled eggplant slices then cut into quarters.
9. Add eggplant to the salad bowl and pour dressing over salad.
10. Toss well.
11. Serve and enjoy.

Cauliflower Radish Salad

Preparation time: 15 minutes

Serves: 4

Ingredients:

- 12 radishes, trimmed and chopped
- 1 tsp dried dill
- 1 tsp Dijon mustard
- 1 tbsp cider vinegar
- 1 tbsp olive oil
- 1 cup parsley, chopped
- ½ medium cauliflower head, trimmed and chopped
- ½ tsp black pepper
- ¼ tsp sea salt

Directions:

1. In a mixing bowl, combine together cauliflower, parsley, and radishes.
2. In a small bowl, whisk together olive oil, dill, mustard, vinegar, pepper, and salt.
3. Pour dressing over salad and toss well.

4. Serve immediately and enjoy.

Citrus Salad

Preparation Time:10 minutes

Cooking Time:0 minute

Servings: 8

Ingredients:

- 3 tbsp. freshly squeezed lemon juice
- 5 tbsp. olive oil
- 2 tsp. Dijon mustard
- 2 tbsp. honey
- 1 tbsp. shallot, minced
- 1 tbsp. fresh thyme, chopped
- Salt and pepper to taste
- 4 cups mixed salad greens
- 2 cups radicchio leaves, shredded
- 3 oranges, sliced
- 1 grapefruit, sliced
- ¼ cup pomegranate seeds

Directions:

1. Combine lemon juice, oil, mustard, honey, shallot, thyme, salt and pepper in a glass jar with lid.
2. Arrange the salad greens and radicchio leaves in a salad bowl.
3. Top with the oranges and grapefruit slices.
4. Sprinkle top with the pomegranate seeds.
5. Serve with the dressing on the side.

Spinach Salad

Preparation Time: 10 minutes

Cooking Time: 0 minutes

Servings: 4

Ingredients:

- 2 tbsp. olive oil
- Salt and pepper to taste
- 4 tsp. vinegar
- 8 cups baby spinach
- 1 cup raspberries
- ¼ cup goat cheese, crumbled
- ¼ cup hazelnuts, toasted and chopped

Directions:

1. Combine the vinegar, salt, pepper and oil in a bowl.
2. Toss the spinach and raspberries in this mixture.
3. Top with the goat cheese and hazelnuts. Lovely

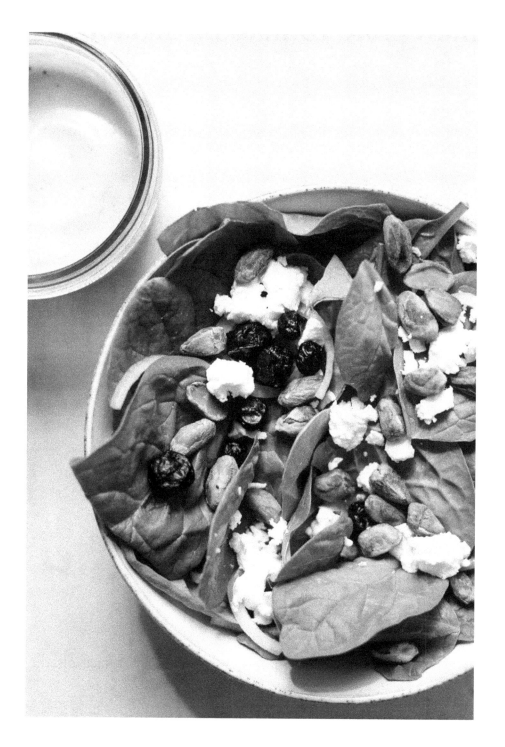

Incredible Tomato Basil Soup

Servings: 6

Preparation time: 6 hours and 10 minutes

Ingredients:

- 1 cup of chopped celery
- 1 cup of chopped carrots
- 74 ounce of whole tomatoes, canned
- 2 cups of chopped white onion
- 2 teaspoons of minced garlic
- 1 tablespoon of salt
- 1/2 teaspoon of ground white pepper
- 1/4 cup of basil leaves and more for garnishing
- 1 bay leaf
- 32 fluid ounce of vegetable broth
- 1/2 cup of grated Parmesan cheese

Directions:

1. Using an 8 quarts or larger slow cooker, place all the ingredients.
2. Stir until itmixes properly and cover the top.

3. Plug in the slow cooker; adjust the cooking time to 5 hours and let it cook on the high heat setting or until the vegetables are tender.

4. Blend the soup with a submersion blender or until soup reaches your desired state.

5. Garnish it with the cheese, basil leaves and serve.

Spinach, Strawberry & Avocado Salad

Preparation Time: 5 minutes

Cooking Time: 0 minute

Servings: 2

Ingredients:

- 6 cups baby spinach
- 1 cup strawberries, sliced
- 2 tbsp. onion, chopped
- ½ avocado, diced
- 4 tbsp. vinaigrette
- 4 tbsp. walnuts, toasted

Directions:

1. Toss the spinach, strawberries, onion and avocado in the vinaigrette.
2. Sprinkle with the walnuts.

Savory Squash & Apple Dish

Servings: 6

Preparation time: 4 hours and 15 minutes

Ingredients:

- 8 ounce of dried cranberries
- 4 medium-sized apples, peeled, cored and chopped
- 3 pounds of butternut squash, peeled, seeded and cubed
- Half of a medium-sized white onion, peeled and diced
- 1 tablespoon of ground cinnamon
- 1 1/2 teaspoons of ground nutmeg

Directions:

1. Take a 6-quarts slow cooker, grease it with a non-stick cooking spray and place the ingredients in it.
2. Stir properly and cover the top.
3. Plug in the slow cooker; adjust the cooking time to 4 hours and let it cook on the low heat setting or until it cooks thoroughly.
4. Serve right away.

Wonderful Steamed Artichoke

Servings: 4

Preparation time: 4 hours and 5 minutes

Ingredients:

- 8 medium-sized artichokes, stemmed and trimmed
- 2 teaspoons of salt
- 4 tablespoons of lemon juice

Directions:

1. Cut 1-inch part of the artichoke from the top and place it in a 6-quarts slow cooker, facing an upright position.
2. Using a bowl, place the lemon juice and pour in the salt until it mixes properly.
3. Pour this mixture over the artichoke and add the water to cover at least ¾ of the artichokes.
4. Cover the top, plug in the slow cooker; adjust the cooking time to 4 hours and let it cook on the high heat setting or until the artichokes get soft.
5. Serve immediately.

Tangy Corn Chowder

Servings: 6

Preparation time: 5 hours and 15 minutes

Ingredients:

- 24 ounce of cooked kernel corn
- 3 medium-sized potatoes, pee led and diced
- 2 red chile peppers, minced
- 1 large white onion, peeled and diced
- 1 teaspoon of minced garlic
- 2 teaspoons of salt
- 1/2 teaspoon of ground black pepper
- 1 tablespoon of red chili powder
- 1 tablespoon of dried parsley
- 1/4 cup of vegan margarine
- 14 fluid ounce of soy milk
- 1 lime, juiced
- 24 fluid ounce of vegetable broth

Directions:

1. Using a 6-quarts slow cooker place all the ingredients except for the soy milk, margarine, and lime juice.
2. Stir properly and cover it with the lid.
3. Then plug in the slow cooker and let it cook for 3 to 4 hours at the high setting or until it is cooked thoroughly.
4. When done, process the mixture with an immersion blender or until it gets smooth.
5. Pour in the milk, margarine and stir properly.
6. Continue cooking the soup for 1 hour at the low heat setting.
7. Drizzle it with the lime juice and serve.

"Potato" Salad

Preparation Time: 10 minutes

Cooking time: 15 minutes

Servings: 4

Ingredients:

- 8 oz turnip, peeled
- 1 carrot, peeled
- 1 bay leaf
- ¼ teaspoon peppercorns
- 1 teaspoon salt
- ½ teaspoon cayenne pepper
- 1 tablespoon fresh parsley, chopped
- 3 eggs, boiled
- 3 tablespoon sour cream
- 1 tablespoon mustard
- 2 cups water, for vegetables

Directions:

1. Put turnip and carrot in the saucepan.

2. Add water, peppercorns, bay leaf, and salt.
3. Close the lid and boil vegetables for 15 minutes over high heat.
4. The cooked vegetables should be tender.
5. Meanwhile, peel eggs and chop them.
6. Put the chopped eggs in the bowl.
7. Sprinkle them with cayenne pepper and chopped parsley.
8. In the separate bowl stir together mustard and sour cream.
9. When the vegetables are cooked, strain them and transfer in the salad bowl.
10. Add mustard sauce and stir.

Chunky Potato Soup

Servings: 6

Preparation time: 6 hours and 10 minutes

Ingredients:

- 1 medium-sized carrot, grated
- 6 medium-sized potatoes, peeled and diced
- 2 stalks of celery, diced
- 1 medium-sized white onion, peeled and diced
- 2 teaspoons of minced garlic
- 1 1/2 teaspoons of salt
- 1 teaspoon of ground black pepper
- 1 1/2 teaspoons of dried sage
- 1 teaspoon of dried thyme
- 2 tablespoons of olive oil
- 2 bay leaves
- 8 1/2 cups of vegetable water

Directions:

1. Using a 6-quarts slow cooker, place all the ingredients and stir properly.

2. Cover it with the lid, plug in the slow cooker and let it cook for 6 hours at the high heat setting or until the potatoes are tender.

3. Serve right away.

Simple Bechamel Sauce

Preparation Time: 30minutes

Servings: 8

Ingredients:

- 3 tablespoons vegan butter
- 2 tablespoons flour
- 2 cups unheated milk
- Season the salt and pepper
- A pinch of nutmeg (optional)

Directions:

1. Melt the butter in a saucepan over medium heat.
2. Add the flour and beat until thick and bubbly but not browned (approximately 2 minutes).
3. Pour the warm milk into the pan and continue stirring until the sauce has thickened (approximately 3 minutes).
4. Add salt, pepper and nutmeg to the pan and stir.
5. Use it immediately or, if done beforehand, put wax paper over the sauce until ready to use.

Spicy Cheese Sauce

Preparation Time: 10minutes

Ingredients:

- 1/2 teaspoon paprika
- 1/4 tsp Chipotle pepper powder
- 1/2 teaspoon sea salt (more to taste)
- 1 teaspoon Cumin (more to taste)

Directions:

1. Put all the INGREDIENTS in a powerful blender.
2. Mix everything smooth and creamy.
3. Adjust the spices to taste and add more water to obtain the desired consistency.

Homemade Worcestershire Sauce

Preparation Time: 30minutes

Ingredients:

- 1 cup apple cider vinegar
- 1/3 cup dark molasses
- 1/4 cup tamari
- 1/4 cup of water
- 3 tablespoons lemon juice
- 1 1/2 tablespoons salt
- 1/2 tablespoon dried mustard powder
- 1 teaspoon onion powder
- 3/4 teaspoon ground ginger
- ½ teaspoon black pepper
- 1/4 teaspoon garlic powder
- 1/4 teaspoon cayenne pepper
- 1/4 teaspoon ground cinnamon
- 1/8 teaspoon ground cloves or allspice
- 1/8 teaspoon ground cardamom

Directions:

1. Mix all the INGREDIENTS in a blender.

2. Pour the mixture into a medium size saucepan and boil.

3. Remove from heat and pour into a sterile beer glass or a clean 12.7 oz beer bottle or cider with a tight lid or lid.

4. Store in the fridge.

5. Let it remain that way for a long time!

Tempeh Finger Fries

Preparation time: 10 minutes

Cooking time: 25 minutes

Servings: 4

Ingredients:

- 8 ounces fry-sliced tempeh
- 1 tbsp. olive oil
- 2 tbsp. soy sauce
- 1 tsp. chili powder

Directions:

1. Begin by heating up the soy sauce and the olive oil together in a skillet for about two minutes.
2. Afterwards, add the sliced tempeh, making sure to coat the tempeh with the sauce.
3. Add the chili powder and stir well.
4. Sauté this mixture well for about seven or eight minutes.
5. The tempeh should be crisp on all sides.
6. Enjoy with your favorite dip!

Freedom Sweet Fries

Preparation time: 10 minutes

Cooking time: 45 minutes

Servings: 4

Ingredients:

- 2 sliced sweet potato fries
- 1 tsp. paprika
- 2 tsp. olive oil
- ½ tsp. cumin
- 1 tsp. salt

Directions:

1. Begin by preheating the oven to 350 degrees Fahrenheit.
2. Next, stir together the sweet potatoes and all of the above ingredients in a large mixing bowl.
3. Make sure to completely coat the sweet potato fries.
4. Next, spread the sweet potato fries out on a baking sheet, and allow them to bake for fifty minutes.
5. Serve warm, and enjoy

Cauliflower Steaks

Serves: 4

Preparation Time: 30 Minutes

Ingredients:

- ¼ Teaspoon Black Pepper
- ½ Teaspoon Sea Salt, Fine
- 1 Tablespoon Olive Oil
- 1 Head Cauliflower, Large
- ¼ Cup Creamy Hummus
- 2 Tablespoons Lemon Sauce
- ½ Cup Peanuts, Crushed (Optional)

Directions:

1. Start by heating your oven to 425.
2. Cut your cauliflower stems, and then remove the leaves.
3. Put the cut side down, and then slice half down the middle.
4. Cut into ¾ inch steaks.
5. If you cut them thinner, they could fall apart.

6. Arrange them in a single layer on a baking sheet, drizzling with oil.
7. Season and bake for twenty to twenty-five minutes.
8. They should be lightly browned and tender.
9. Spread your hummus on the steaks, drizzling with your lemon sauce.
10. Top with peanuts if you're using it.

Interesting Facts:

Cauliflower: This vegetable is an extremely high source of vitamin A, vitamin B1, B2 and B3.

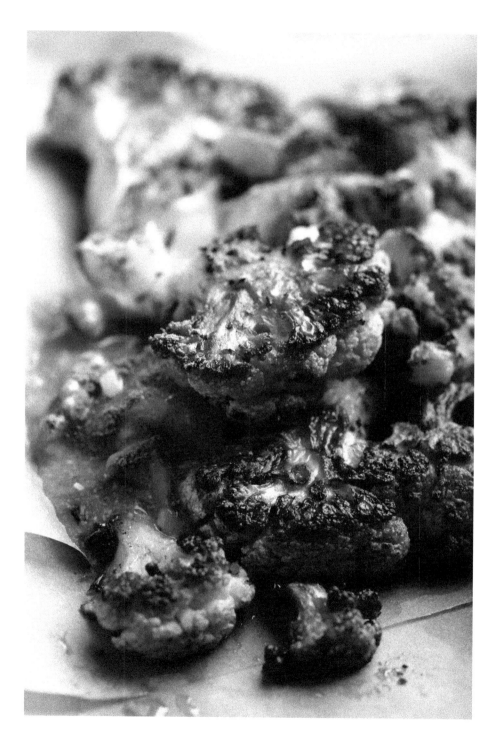

Tofu & Asparagus Stir Fry

Serves: 3 Time: 20 Minutes

Ingredients:

- 1 Tablespoon Ginger, Peeled & Grated
- 8 Ounces Firm Tofu, Chopped into Slices
- 4 Green Onions, Sliced Thin Toasted Sesame Oil to Taste
- 1 Bunch Asparagus, Trimmed & Chopped
- 1 Handful Cashew Nuts, Chopped & Toasted
- 2 Tablespoons Hoisin Sauce
- 1 Lime, Juiced & Zested
- 1 Handful Mint, Fresh & Chopped
- 1 Handful Basil, Fresh & Chopped
- 3 Cloves Garlic, Chopped
- 3 Handfuls Spinach, Chopped
- Pinch Sea Salt

Directions:

1. Get out a wok and heat up your oil.
2. Add in your tofu, cooking for a few minutes.

3. Put your tofu to the side, and then sauté your red pepper flakes, ginger, salt, onions and asparagus for a minute.

4. Mix in your spinach, garlic, and cashews, cooking for another two minutes.

5. Add your tofu back in, and then drizzle in your lime juice, lime zest, hoisin sauce, cooking for another half a minute.

6. Remove it from heat, adding in your mint and basil.

Interesting Facts: Sesame seeds can be easily added to crackers, bread, salads, and stir-fry meals. Bonus: Help in lowering cholesterol and high blood pressure.

Double bonus: Help with asthma, arthritis, and migraines!

Mexican Lentil Soup

Preparation time: 5 minutes

Cooking time: 45 minutes

Servings: 6

Ingredients:

- 2 cups green lentils
- 1 medium red bell pepper, cored, diced
- 1 medium white onion, peeled, diced
- 2 cups diced tomatoes
- 8 ounces diced green chilies
- 2 celery stalks, diced
- 2 medium carrots, peeled, diced
- 1 ½ teaspoon minced garlic
- 1/2 teaspoon salt
- 1 tablespoon cumin
- 1/4 teaspoon smoked paprika
- 1 teaspoon oregano
- 1/8 teaspoon hot sauce
- 2 tablespoons olive oil
- 8 cups vegetable broth

- ¼ cup cilantro, for garnish
- 1 avocado, peeled, pitted, diced, for garnish

Directions:

1. Take a large pot over medium heat, add oil and when hot, add all the vegetables, reserving tomatoes and chilies, and cook for 5 minutes until softened.
2. Then add garlic, stir in oregano, cumin, and paprika, and continue cooking for 1 minute.
3. Add lentils, tomatoes and green chilies, season with salt, pour in the broth and simmer the soup for 40 minutes until cooked.
4. When done, ladle soup into bowls, top with avocado and cilantro and serve straight away

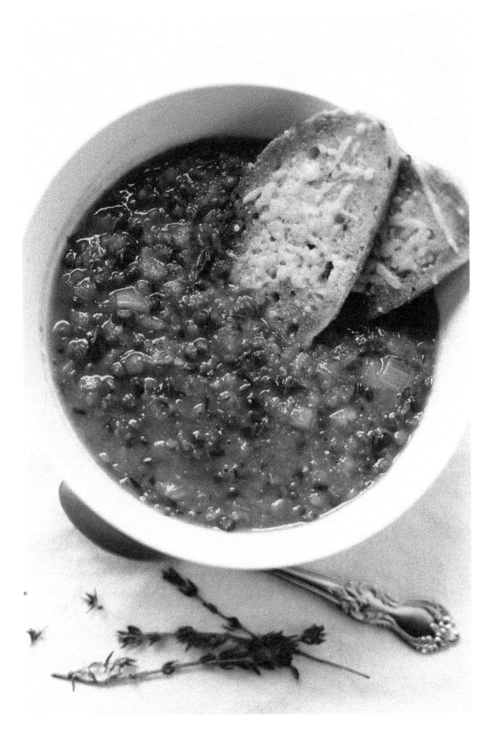

Cauliflower Soup

Preparation time: 10 minutes

Cooking time: 40 minutes

Servings: 2

Ingredients:

- 1 small head of cauliflower, cut into florets
- 4 tablespoons pomegranate seeds
- 2 sprigs of thyme and more for garnishing
- 1 teaspoon minced garlic
- 2/3 teaspoon salt
- 1/3 teaspoon ground black pepper
- 1 tablespoon olive oil
- 1 1/2 cups vegetable stock
- 1/2 cup coconut milk, unsweetened

Directions:

1. Take a pot, place it over medium heat, add oil and when hot, add garlic and cook for 1 minute until fragrant.
2. Add florets, thyme, pour in the stock and bring the mixture to boil.

3. Switch heat to the medium low level, simmer the soup for 30 minutes until florets are tender, then remove the pot from heat, discard the thyme and puree using an immersion blender until smooth.

4. Stir milk into the soup, season with salt and black pepper, then garnish with pomegranate seeds and thyme sprigs and serve.

Asparagus Soup

Preparation time: 10 minutes

Cooking time: 20 minutes

Servings: 4

Ingredients:

- 1/2 head of medium cauliflower, cut into florets
- 1 medium white onion, peeled, sliced
- 2 pounds asparagus, ends trimmed, chopped
- 2 teaspoons minced garlic
- ½ teaspoon ground black pepper
- 1/2 cup nutritional yeast
- ½ teaspoon salt
- 1 lemon, juiced
- 1 tablespoon olive oil
- 6 cups vegetable broth

Directions:

1. Take a large stockpot, place it over medium-high heat, add oil and when hot, add onions and garlic, and cook for 7 minutes until onions are translucent.

2. Then add cauliflower florets and asparagus, pour in vegetable broth, bring to boil, then switch heat to medium level and simmer for 10 minutes until vegetables are tender.

3. Puree soup by using an immersion blender, then return it over medium heat, season with salt and black pepper, stir in lemon juice and yeast and serve straight away.

Butternut Squash and Coconut Milk

Soup Preparation time: 10 minutes

Cooking time: 35 minutes

Servings: 6

Ingredients:

- 1 cup diced parsnips
- 2 cups diced sweet potato
- 1 large sweet onion, peeled, diced
- 1 ½ cups diced carrots
- 4 cups diced butternut squash
- 2 teaspoons minced garlic
- 1/4 teaspoon ground ginger
- ¼ teaspoon ground black pepper
- ½ teaspoon of sea salt
- 1/4 teaspoon ground allspice
- 1 teaspoon poultry seasoning
- 1 teaspoon pumpkin pie spice
- 1/4 teaspoon ground cinnamon
- 32 ounces vegetable stock

- 14 ounces coconut milk, unsweetened

Directions:

1. Take a large Dutch oven, place it over medium heat, add onions, drizzle with 2 tablespoons water and cook for 5 minutes until softened, drizzling with more 2 tablespoons at a time if required.
2. Then stir in garlic, cook for another minute, switch heat to the high level, add remaining ingredients, reserving milk, salt, and black pepper, and bring the soup to boil.
3. Then switch heat to medium-low level and simmer for 20 minutes until vegetables are tender.
4. When done, puree soup by using an immersion blender, then stir in coconut milk, season with salt and black pepper and cook for 3 minutes until warm.
5. Serve straight away

Potato and Kale Soup

Preparation time: 5 minutes

Cooking time: 15 minutes

Servings: 2

Ingredients:

- 1 small white onion, peeled, chopped
- 2 ½ cups cubed potatoes
- 2 cups leek, cut into rings
- 1/2 cup chopped carrots
- 1/2 cup chopped celery
- ½ teaspoon minced garlic
- 2/3 teaspoon salt
- 1/3 teaspoon ground black pepper
- 1 tablespoon olive oil
- 3 1/2 cups vegetable broth
- 1 cup kale, cut into stripes
- Croutons, for serving

Directions:

1. Take a large pot, place it over medium heat, add oil and when hot, add onion and cook for 2 minutes until sauté.
2. Stir in garlic, cook for another minute, then add all the vegetables and continue cooking for 3 minutes.
3. Pour in broth, cook for 15 minutes, then add kale and cook for 2 minutes until tender.
4. Season soup with salt and black pepper, puree by using an immersion blender until smooth, then top with croutons and serve.

Roasted Cauliflower Soup

Preparation time: 10 minutes

Cooking time: 60 minutes

Servings: 4

Ingredients:

- 1 medium head of cauliflower, cut into florets
- 1 small white onion, peeled, diced
- 1 medium carrot, peeled, diced
- 1 stalk of celery, diced
- 1 head of garlic, top off
- 2/3 teaspoon salt
- 1/3 teaspoon ground black pepper
- 1 teaspoon smoked paprika
- 2 tablespoons nutritional yeast
- 1 teaspoon hot smoked paprika
- 4 tablespoons olive oil
- 12 ounces coconut milk, unsweetened
- 4 cups vegetable broth
- ½ cup chopped parsley

Directions:

1. Switch on the oven, then set it to 400 degrees F and let it preheat.

2. Place top off garlic on a piece of foil, drizzle with 1 tablespoon oil, and then wrap.

3. Place cauliflower florets in a bowl, drizzle with 2 tablespoons oil, season with salt and black pepper, and toss until well coated.

4. Take a baking sheet, spread cauliflower florets in it in a single layer, add wrapped garlic and bake for 30 minutes until roasted.

5. Then place a large pot over medium-high heat, add remaining oil and when hot, add onions and cook for 3 minutes.

6. Then add celery and carrot, continue cooking for 3 minutes, season with salt and paprika, pour in broth, and bring it to a boil.

7. Add roasted garlic and florets, bring the mixture to boil, then switch heat to medium-low level and simmer for 15 minutes.

8. Puree the soup by using an immersion blender, stir in milk and yeast until mixed and simmer for 3 minutes until hot.

9. Garnish soup with parsley and then serve.

Ramen Noodle Soup

Preparation time: 10 minutes

Cooking time: 20 minutes

Servings: 2

Ingredients:

For The Mushrooms and Tofu:

- 2 cups sliced shiitake mushrooms
- 6 ounces tofu, extra-firm, drained, sliced
- 1 tablespoon olive oil
- 1 tablespoon soy sauce

For the Noodle Soup:

- 2 packs of dried ramen noodles
- 1 medium carrot, peeled, grated
- 1 inch of ginger, grated
- 1 teaspoon minced garlic
- ¾ cup baby spinach leaves
- 1 tablespoon olive oil
- 6 cups vegetable broth

For Garnish:

- Sesame seeds as needed
- Soy sauce as needed
- Sriracha sauce as needed

Directions:

1. Prepare mushrooms and tofu and for this, place tofu pieces in a plastic bag, add soy sauce, seal the bag and turn it upside until tofu is coated.
2. Take a skillet pan, place it over medium heat, add oil and when hot, add tofu slices and cook for 5 to 10 minutes until crispy and browned on all sides, flipping frequently and when done, set aside until required.
3. Add mushrooms into the pan, cook for 8 minutes until golden, pour soy sauce from tofu pieces in it, and stir until coated.
4. Meanwhile, prepare noodle soup and for this, take a soup pot, place it over medium-high heat, add oil and when hot, add garlic and ginger and cook for 1 minute until fragrant.
5. Then pour in the broth, bring the mixture to boil, add noodles and cook until tender.
6. Then stir spinach into the noodle soup, remove the pot from heat and distribute evenly between bowls.

7. Add mushrooms and tofu along with garnishing and then serve.

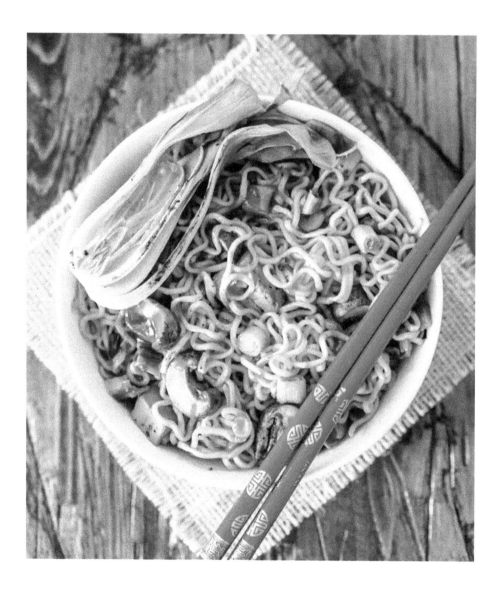

Hot and Sour Soup

Preparation time: 5 minutes

Cooking time: 20 minutes

Servings: 4

Ingredients:

- 2 tablespoons dried wood ears
- 3.5 ounces bamboo shoots, sliced into thin strips
- 1 medium carrot, peeled, sliced into thin strips
- 5 dried shiitake mushrooms
- 1 tablespoon grated ginger
- 1 teaspoon minced garlic
- 1 teaspoon ground black pepper
- 1 teaspoon salt
- 1/4 cup soy sauce
- 1 teaspoon sugar
- 1/2 cup rice vinegar
- 4 cups vegetable stock
- 1 1/2 cup water, boiling
- 7.5 ounces tofu, extra-firm, drained
- 1 tablespoon green onion tops, chopped

- ¼ cup water, at room temperature
- 2 tablespoons cornstarch
- 1 teaspoon sesame oil

Directions:

1. Take a small bowl, place wood ears in it, then pour in boiling water until covered and let stand for 30 minutes.
2. Meanwhile, take another bowl, place mushrooms in it, pour in 1 ½ cup water and let the mushrooms stand for 30 minutes.
3. After 30 minutes, drain the wood ears, rinse well and cut into slices, remove and discard the hard bits.
4. Similarly, drain the mushrooms, reserving their soaking liquid and slice the mushrooms, removing and discarding their stems.
5. Take a large pot, place it over medium-high heat, add all the ingredients including reserved mushroom liquid, leave the last five ingredients, stir well and bring the mixture to boil.
6. Then switch heat to medium level and simmer the soup for 10 minutes until cooked.
7. Meanwhile, place cornstarch in a bowl, add water at room temperature, and stir well until smooth.

8. Cut tofu into 1-inch pieces, add into the simmering soup along with cornstarch mixture, and continue to simmer the soup until it reaches to desired thickness.

9. Drizzle with sesame oil, distribute soup into bowls, garnish with green onions and serve.

Thai Coconut Soup

Preparation time: 10 minutes

Cooking time: 15 minutes

Servings: 12

Ingredients:

- 2 mangos, peeled, cut into bite-size pieces
- 1/2 cup green lentils, cooked
- 2 sweet potatoes, peeled, cubed
- 1/2 cup quinoa, cooked
- 1 green bell pepper, cored, cut into strips
- ½ teaspoon chopped basil
- ½ teaspoon chopped rosemary
- 2 tablespoons red curry paste
- 1/4 cup mixed nut
- 2 teaspoons orange zest
- 30 ounces coconut milk, unsweetened

Directions:

1. Take a large saucepan, place it over medium-high heat, add sweet potatoes, pour in the milk and bring the mixture to boil.

2. Then switch heat to medium-low level, add remaining ingredients, except for quinoa and lentils, stir and cook for 15 minutes until vegetables have softened.

3. Then stir in quinoa and lentils, cook for 3 minutes until hot, and then serve.

Pomegranate and Walnut Stew

Preparation time: 10 minutes

Cooking time: 55 minutes

Servings: 6

Ingredients:

- 1 head of cauliflower, cut into florets
- 1 medium white onion, peeled, diced
- 1 1/2 cups California walnuts, toasted
- 1 cup yellow split peas
- 1 1/2 tablespoons honey
- ¼ teaspoon salt
- ½ teaspoon turmeric
- ½ teaspoon cinnamon
- 2 tablespoons olive oil, separated
- 4 cups pomegranate juice
- 2 tablespoons chopped parsley
- 2 tablespoons chopped walnuts, for garnishing

Directions:

1. Take a medium saute pan, place it over medium heat, add walnuts, cook for 5 minutes until toasted and then cool for 5 minutes.

2. Transfer walnuts to the food processor, pulse for 2 minutes until ground, and set aside until required.

3. Take a large saute pan, place it over medium heat, add 1 tablespoon oil and when hot, add onion and cook for 5 minutes until softened.

4. Switch heat to medium-low heat, then add lentils and walnuts, stir in cinnamon, salt, and turmeric, pour in honey and pomegranate, stir until mixed and simmer the mixture for 40 minutes until the sauce has reduced by half and lentils have softened.

5. Meanwhile, place cauliflower florets in a food processor and then pulse for 2 minutes until mixture resembles rice.

6. Take a medium to saute pan, place it over medium heat, add remaining oil and when hot, add cauliflower rice, cook for 5 minutes until softened, and then season with salt.

7. Serve cooked pomegranate and walnut sauce with cooked cauliflower rice and garnish with walnuts and parsley.

Vegetarian Irish Stew

Preparation time: 5 minutes

Cooking time: 38 minutes

Servings: 6

Ingredients:

- 1 cup textured vegetable protein, chunks
- ½ cup split red lentils
- 2 medium onions, peeled, sliced
- 1 cup sliced parsnip
- 2 cups sliced mushrooms
- 1 cup diced celery,
- 1/4 cup flour
- 4 cups vegetable stock
- 1 cup rutabaga
- 1 bay leaf
- ½ cup fresh parsley
- 1 teaspoon sugar
- ¼ teaspoon ground black pepper
- 1/4 cup soy sauce
- ¼ teaspoon thyme

- 2 teaspoons marmite
- ¼ teaspoon rosemary
- 2/3 teaspoon salt
- ¼ teaspoon marjoram

Directions:

1. Take a large soup pot, place it over medium heat, add oil and when it gets hot, add onions and cook for 5 minutes until softened.
2. Then switch heat to the low level, sprinkle with flour, stir well, add remaining ingredients, stir until combined and simmer for 30 minutes until vegetables have cooked.
3. When done, season the stew with salt and black pepper and then serve.

Spinach and Cannellini Bean Stew

Preparation time: 10 minutes

Cooking time: 15 minutes

Servings: 6

Ingredients:

- 28 ounces cooked cannellini beans
- 24 ounces tomato passata
- 17 ounces spinach chopped
- ¼ teaspoon ground black pepper
- 2/3 teaspoon salt
- 1 ¼ teaspoon curry powder
- 1 cup cashew butter
- ¼ teaspoon cardamom
- 2 tablespoons olive oil
- 1 teaspoon salt
- ¼ cup cashews
- 2 tablespoons chopped basil
- 2 tablespoons chopped parsley

Directions:

1. Take a large saucepan, place it over medium heat, add 1 tablespoon oil and when hot, add spinach and cook for 3 minutes until fried.
2. Then stir in butter and tomato passata until well mixed, bring the mixture to a near boil, add beans and season with ¼ teaspoon curry powder, black pepper, and salt.
3. Take a small saucepan, place it over medium heat, add remaining oil, stir in cashew, stir in salt and curry powder and cook for 4 minutes until roasted, set aside until required.
4. Transfer cooked stew into a bowl, top with roasted cashews, basil, and parsley, and then serve.

Cabbage Stew

Preparation time: 10 minutes

Cooking time: 50 minutes

Servings: 6

Ingredients:

- 12 ounces cooked Cannellini beans
- 8 ounces smoked tofu, firm, sliced
- 1 medium cabbage, chopped
- 1 large white onion, peeled, julienned
- 2 ½ teaspoon minced garlic
- 1 tablespoon sweet paprika
- 5 tablespoons tomato paste
- 3 teaspoons smoked paprika
- 1/3 teaspoon ground black pepper
- 2 teaspoons dried thyme
- 2/3 teaspoon salt
- ½ tsp ground coriander
- 3 bay leaves
- 4 tablespoons olive oil
- 1 cup vegetable broth

Directions:

1. Take a large saucepan, place it over medium heat, add 3 tablespoons oil and when hot, add onion and garlic and cook for 3 minutes or until saute.

2. Add cabbage, pour in water, simmer for 10 minutes or until softened, then stir in all the spices and continue cooking for 30 minutes.

3. Add beans and tomato paste, pour in water, stir until mixed and cook for 15 minutes until thoroughly cooked.

4. Take a separate skillet pan, add 1 tablespoon oil and when hot, add tofu slices and cook for 5 minutes until golden brown on both sides.

5. Serve cooked cabbage stew with fried tofu.

African Peanut Lentil Soup

Preparation time: 10 minutes

Cooking time: 25 minutes

Servings: 3

Ingredients:

- 1/2 cup red lentils
- 1/2 medium white onion, sliced
- 2 medium tomatoes, chopped
- 1/2 cup baby spinach
- 1/2 cup sliced zucchini
- 1/2 cup sliced sweet potatoes
- ½ cup sliced potatoes
- ½ cup broccoli florets
- 2 teaspoons minced garlic
- 1 inch of ginger, grated
- 1 tablespoon tomato paste
- 1/4 teaspoon ground black pepper
- 1 teaspoon salt
- 1 ½ teaspoon ground cumin
- 2 teaspoons ground coriander

- 2 tablespoons peanuts
- 1 teaspoon Harissa Spice Blend
- 1 tablespoon sambal oelek
- 1/4 cup almond butter
- 1 teaspoon olive oil
- 1 teaspoon lemon juice
- 2 ½ cups vegetable stock

Directions:

1. Take a large saucepan, place it over medium heat, add oil and when hot, add onion and cook for 5 minutes until translucent.
2. Meanwhile, place tomatoes in a blender, add garlic, ginger and sambal oelek along with all the spices and pulse until pureed.
3. Pour this mixture into the onions, cook for 5 minutes, then add remaining ingredients except for spinach, peanuts and lemon juice and simmer for 15 minutes.
4. Taste to adjust the seasoning, stir in spinach, and cook for 5 minutes until cooked.
5. Ladle soup into bowls, garnish with lime juice and peanuts and serve.

Eggplant, Onion and Tomato Stew

Preparation time: 5 minutes

Cooking time: 5 minutes

Servings: 4

Ingredients:

- 3 1/2 cups cubed eggplant
- 1 cup diced white onion
- 2 cups diced tomatoes
- 1 teaspoon ground cumin
- 1/8 teaspoon ground cayenne pepper
- 1 teaspoon salt
- 1 cup tomato sauce
- 1/2 cup water

Directions:

1. Switch on the instant pot, place all the ingredients in it, stir until mixed, and seal the pot.

2. Press the 'manual' button and cook for 5 minutes at high-pressure setting until cooked.
3. When done, do quick pressure release, open the instant pot, and stir the stew.
4. Serve straight away.

Brussel Sprouts Stew

Preparation time: 10 minutes

Cooking time: 55 minutes

Servings: 4

Ingredients:

- 35 ounces Brussels sprouts
- 5 medium potato, peeled, chopped
- 1 medium onion, peeled, chopped
- 2 carrot, peeled, cubed
- 2 teaspoon smoked paprika
- 1/8 teaspoon ground black pepper
- 1/8 teaspoon salt
- 3 tablespoons caraway seeds
- 1/2 teaspoon red chili powder
- 1 tablespoon nutmeg 1 tablespoon olive oil
- 4 ½ cups hot vegetable stock

Directions:

1. Take a large pot, place it over medium-high heat, add oil and when hot, add onion and cook for 1 minute.
2. Then add carrot and potato, cook for 2 minutes, then add Brussel sprouts and cook for 5 minutes.
3. Stir in all the spices, pour in vegetable stock, bring the mixture to boil, switch heat to medium-low and simmer for 45 minutes until cooked and stew reach to desired thickness.
4. Serve straight away.

Black Bean and Quinoa Stew

Preparation time: 10 minutes

Cooking time: 6 hours

Servings: 6

Ingredients:

- 1 pound black beans, dried, soaked overnight
- 3/4 cup quinoa, uncooked
- 1 medium red bell pepper, cored, chopped
- 1 medium red onion, peeled, diced
- 1 medium green bell pepper, cored, chopped
- 28-ounce diced tomatoes
- 2 dried chipotle peppers
- 1 ½ teaspoon minced garlic
- 2/3 teaspoon sea salt
- 2 teaspoons red chili powder
- 1/3 teaspoon ground black pepper
- 1 teaspoon coriander powder
- 1 dried cinnamon stick
- 1/4 cup cilantro
- 7 cups of water

Directions:

1. Switch on the slow cooker, add all the ingredients in it, except for salt, and stir until mixed.
2. Shut the cooker with lid and cook for 6 hours at a high heat setting until cooked.
3. When done, stir salt into the stew until mixed, remove cinnamon sticks and serve

Portobello Mushroom Stew

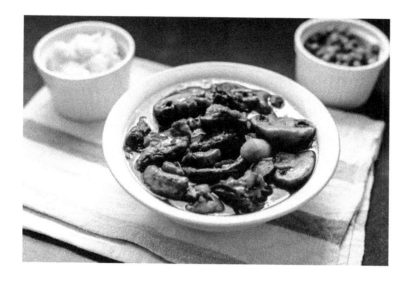

Preparation time: 10 minutes

Cooking time: 8 hours

Servings: 4

Ingredients:

- 8 cups vegetable broth
- 1 cup dried wild mushrooms
- 1 cup dried chickpeas
- 3 cups chopped potato
- 2 cups chopped carrots
- 1 cup corn kernels

- 2 cups diced white onions
- 1 tablespoon minced parsley
- 3 cups chopped zucchini
- 1 tablespoon minced rosemary
- 1 1/2 teaspoon ground black pepper
- 1 teaspoon dried sage
- 2/3 teaspoon salt
- 1 teaspoon dried oregano
- 3 tablespoons soy sauce
- 1 1/2 teaspoons liquid smoke
- 8 ounces tomato paste

Directions:

1. Switch on the slow cooker, add all the ingredients in it, and stir until mixed.
2. Shut the cooker with lid and cook for 10 hours at a high heat setting until cooked.
3. Serve straight away.

Nutrition Value:

Calories: 447 | Cal Fat: 36 g | Carbs: 24 g | Protein: 11 g | Fiber: 2 g

Greens Salad with Black Eyed Peas

Preparation time: 5 minutes

Cooking time: 6 minutes

Servings: 3

Ingredients:

- 2 cups cooked black-eyed peas, cooked
- 1/2 cup cooked quinoa
- 3 cups chopped purple cabbage
- 5 cups chopped kale
- 1/2 of a shallot, peeled, chopped
- 1 1/2 cup shredded carrot
- 1 teaspoon minced garlic
- 1/2 teaspoon sea salt
- 1/3 teaspoon ground black pepper
- 1 tablespoon apple cider vinegar and more as needed
- 1 tablespoon lemon juice
- 2 tablespoons olive oil

Directions:

1. Sauté garlic, shallot, and cabbage in 1 tablespoon for 2 minutes over medium heat, then add remaining oil along with kale, season with salt, and cook for 4 minutes until kale has wilted.
2. Transfer the vegetables to a bowl, add remaining ingredients and toss until combined.
3. Serve straight away

Cranberry and Quinoa Salad

Preparation time: 15 minutes

Cooking time: 0 minute

Servings: 6

Ingredients:

- 2 cups cooked quinoa
- 1/4 cup chopped red onion
- 1/2 cup shredded carrots
- 1/2 cup dried cranberries
- 1/2 cup diced green bell pepper
- 4 tablespoons chopped cilantro
- 1 ½ teaspoon curry powder
- 2/3 teaspoon salt
- 1/3 teaspoon ground black pepper
- 1/8 teaspoon cumin
- 1/3 cup toasted sliced almonds
- 4 tablespoons pepitas
- Olive oil as needed for drizzling
- 1 lime, juiced
- Lime, sliced into wedges

Directions:

1. Place all the ingredients in a large bowl, toss until well combined and let the salad refrigerate for 15 minutes.

2. Serve straight away.

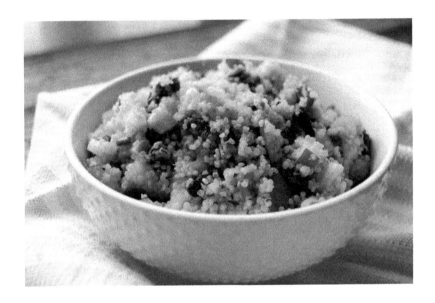

Cucumber Salad with Tofu

Preparation time: 10 minutes

Cooking time: 10 minutes

Servings: 4

Ingredients:

- 2 large cucumbers, sliced
- ½ of medium green bell pepper, sliced into strips
- 14 ounces tofu, extra-firm, drained, cubed
- 3 green onions, chopped
- ½ of green chili pepper, deseeded, sliced into thin strips
- 3 large carrots, shaved into ribbons
- ¼ teaspoon salt
- 1/3 cup roasted almond slices
- 1/2 cup cilantro leaves and stem
- 1 tablespoon sesame oil

For the Dressing:

- 2 cloves of garlic, peeled 1-inch piece of ginger, grated
- ¼ teaspoon red pepper flakes
- 1 tablespoon soy sauce
- 2 tablespoons rice vinegar

- 1 teaspoon maple syrup
- 6 tablespoons sesame oil

Directions:

1. Fry tofu cubes in hot sesame oil over medium heat for 10 minutes until browned and then set aside.
2. Meanwhile, sprinkle salt over cucumber slices, set aside for 10 minutes, then drain them, rinse them and pat dry with paper towels.
3. Prepare the dressing, and for this, place all its ingredients in a food processor and process for 2 minutes until smooth.
4. Place everything in a large bowl, toss until well coated, then top the salad with extra nuts and green onions and serve.

Kidney Beans, Quinoa, Vegetable and Salsa Bowl

Preparation time: 5 minutes

Cooking time: 20 minutes

Servings: 2

Ingredients:

For the Kidney Beans:

- 1 ½ cups cooked kidney beans
- 3/4 teaspoon salt
- 1 large tomato
- 3 cloves of garlic, peeled
- 1/2 teaspoon onion powder
- 1/2 inch piece of ginger
- 1/2 teaspoon paprika
- 1/2 teaspoon dried fenugreek leaves
- 1/3 teaspoon red chili powder
- 1/4 teaspoon turmeric
- 1 teaspoon coriander powder
- 1/2 teaspoon garam masala
- 1/2 teaspoon cumin powder

- 1 teaspoon lemon juice
- 1/2 cup water

For the Vegetables:

- Sliced roasted zucchini as needed
- Sliced roasted broccoli stems as needed
- Sliced radishes as needed
- Sliced lettuce as needed
- Mango salsa as needed

Directions:

1. Prepare the beans, and for this, place all the ingredients, except the first two ones, in a blender, pulse until smooth, then add this mixture into a saucepan and cook for 7 minutes over medium heat until thickened.
2. Then stir in beans, season with salt, and cook for 12 minutes until beans are very tender.
3. When done, place beans in a large bowl, top with vegetables and salsa, toss until mixed and serve

Rainbow Salad Bowl

Preparation time: 10 minutes

Cooking time: 0 minute

Servings: 4

Ingredients:

- 1 cup cooked quinoa
- 1 tablespoon hemp seeds
- 1 head of romaine lettuce, rib removed, leaves chopped
- 1/2 avocado, peeled, pitted, sliced
- ¼ of pickled red onion
- 1/2 cup diced cucumber
- ¼ cup pomegranate seeds
- ½ of lime, juiced
- 1/2 cup cilantro lime hummus

Directions:

1. Place all the ingredients except for lime juice, hummus, and hemp seeds in a bowl and toss until mixed.
2. Place hummus in the middle, drizzle with lime juice, sprinkle with hemp seeds, and then serve.

Lentil Salad With Spinach

Preparation time: 10 minutes

Cooking time: 0 minute

Servings: 4

Ingredients:

For the Salad:

- 2 small apples, cut into small pieces
- 3 cups cooked brown lentils
- ½ cup fresh spinach
- 1/2 cup walnuts, chopped
- 1 medium avocado, pitted, cut into slices
- 1 pomegranate, halved, seeded, rinsed

For the dressing:

- 1 clove of garlic, peeled
- ¼ teaspoon ground black pepper
- ¼ teaspoon salt
- 2 teaspoons orange zest
- 3 tablespoons tahini
- 2 tablespoons olive oil

- 4 tablespoons orange juice
- 6 tablespoons water

Directions:

1. Prepare the dressing, and for this, place all of its ingredients in a food processor and pulse until smooth.
2. Prepare the salad and for this, place all its ingredients in a bowl, toss until mixed, then drizzle with prepared dressing and stir until combined.
3. Serve straight away.

Grilled Corn Salad Bowl

Preparation time: 10 minutes

Cooking time: 0 minute

Servings: 4

Ingredients:

- ½ cup of beluga lentils, cooked
- 2 ears of fresh corn, grilled
- ½ cup pickled onions 1 medium avocado, peeled, sliced
- 1 green chili, chopped
- 2 cups arugula
- ¼ teaspoon ground black pepper
- 2/3 teaspoon salt
- 2 limes, juiced
- 4 tablespoons olive oil
- 10 basil leaves, chopped
- ¼ cup pine nuts, toasted

Directions:

1. Place all the ingredients in the bowl, except for lime juice and oil, and stir until mixed.
2. Drizzle with lime juice and oil, toss until mixed and serve.

Roasted Butternut Squash Salad

Preparation time: 10 minutes

Cooking time: 30 minutes

Servings: 4

Ingredients:

For the Dressing:

- 1/8 teaspoon salt
- 2 tablespoons lime juice
- 1 tablespoon olive oil
- 1 teaspoon sriracha
- 1/2 teaspoon honey

For the Salad:

- 4 cups arugula
- 1 pound butternut squash, peeled, cubed
- 1 1/2 teaspoons olive oil
- 3/4 cups cooked black beans
- 1/4 teaspoon ground black pepper
- 1/4 teaspoon salt
- 1/2 teaspoon ground cumin

- 1/4 cup pepitas, toasted

Directions:

1. Place squash cubes on a baking tray, drizzle with oil, season with salt, black pepper, and cumin, toss until coated and bake for 30 minutes until roasted.
2. Meanwhile, prepare the dressing and for this, place all of its ingredients in a bowl and whisk until smooth.
3. When squash is done, let it cool for 10 minutes, then place it in a bowl along with remaining ingredients of the salad, drizzle with dressing and toss until mixed.
4. Serve straight away.

BBQ Chickpea Salad

Preparation time: 10 minutes

Cooking time: 10 minutes

Servings: 2

Ingredients:

- 2 cups cooked chickpeas
- 1 cup frozen corn kernel
- ¼ of medium red onion, sliced
- 1 cup cherry tomatoes, halved
- 6 cups chopped romaine lettuce
- 1 cup cucumber, sliced
- 6 Tablespoons Ranch Dressing
- 1/2 cup vegan BBQ sauce
- Lime wedges for garnish

Directions:

1. Simmer chickpeas in the BBQ sauce for 10 minutes until chickpeas are glazed with it.

2. Then divide remaining ingredients between two bowls, top with chickpeas, drizzle with dressing and serve with lime wedges.

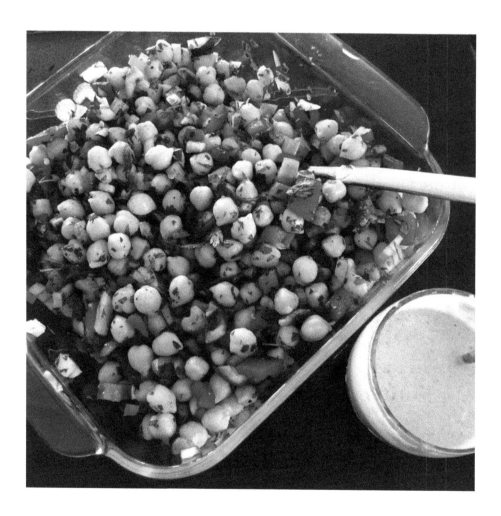

Butternut Squash Quinoa Salad

Preparation time: 10 minutes

Cooking time: 25 minutes

Servings: 4

Ingredients:

For the Salad:

- 1 cup quinoa, cooked
- 3 cups butternut squash, chopped
- 1/3 cup dried cranberries
- 1/3 cup chopped red onion
- 2/3 teaspoon salt
- 1/3 teaspoon ground black pepper
- 3 tablespoons toasted pumpkin seeds
- 1 tablespoon olive oil

For the Dressing:

- ½ teaspoon minced garlic
- 1/3 teaspoon salt
- 1/3 teaspoon ground black pepper
- 1 teaspoon honey

- 1/4 cup balsamic vinegar
- 1 teaspoon Dijon mustard
- 1/2 cup olive oil

Directions:

1. Spread butternut squash on a baking sheet, drizzle with oil, season with black pepper and salt and bake for 25 minutes until roasted and tender.
2. Meanwhile, prepare the dressing and for this, place all of its ingredients in a bowl and whisk until smooth.
3. When done, let squash for 10 minutes, then place them in a bowl, add remaining ingredients for the salad in it, drizzle with dressing and toss until coated.
4. Refrigerate the salad for a minimum of 2 hours and then serve.

Cobb Salad

Preparation time: 10 minutes

Cooking time: 0 minute

Servings: 4

Ingredients:

For the Salad:

- 1/2 cup cooked red beans
- 1/2 cup cooked corn
- 1 medium head of romaine lettuce, shredded
- 1/2 cup chopped tempeh bacon
- 1/2 cup diced tomatoes
- 1/2 cup diced avocado
- 1/2 cup cashews, unsalted

For the Dressing:

- 1 teaspoon garlic powder
- 2 tablespoons lemon juice
- 3 tablespoons soy sauce
- 2 tablespoons cider vinegar
- 1/4 cup agave syrup

- 2 tablespoons Dijon mustard
- 1/4 cup olive oil
- 1/4 cup water

Directions:

1. Prepare the dressing, and for this, place all of its ingredients in a food processor and pulse until smooth.
2. Place all the ingredients for the salad in a large dish, arrange each ingredients in a row, and then drizzle with prepared dressing.
3. Serve straight away.

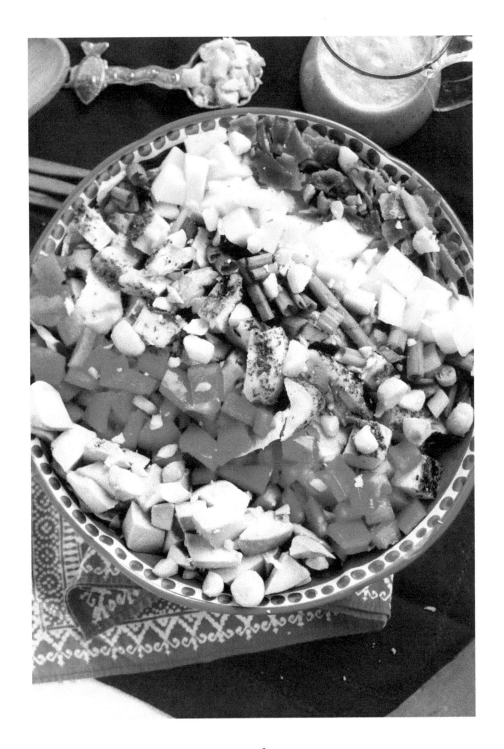

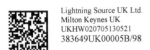

Lightning Source UK Ltd.
Milton Keynes UK
UKHW020705130521
383649UK00005B/98

9 781802 772661